Recognizing Signs of Autism Spectrum Disorder
And
Utilizing Effective Communication with Low Income Parents

A Training Program for Healthcare Providers

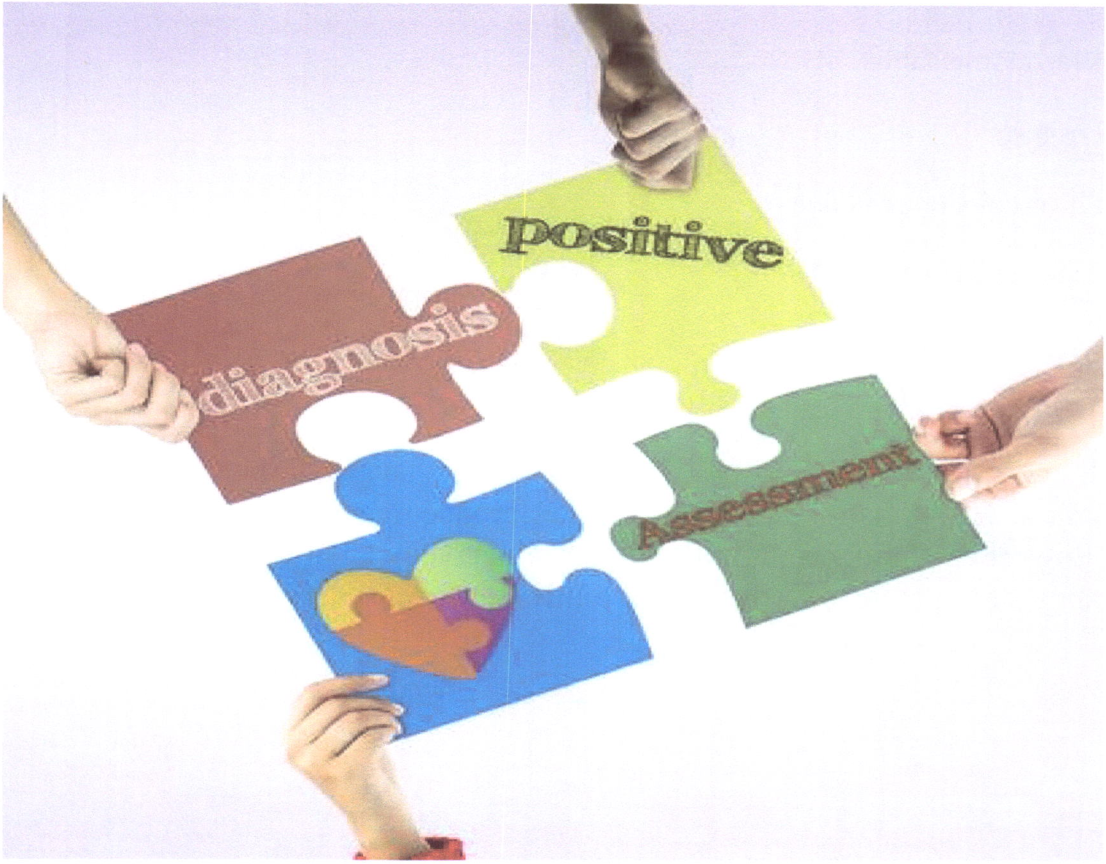

I0494533

How to Use This Booklet

This is a training program designed to be used a learning tool for Healthcare Providers at their leisure.

1. It is comprised of two sets of PowerPoint slides printed in this book and may also be viewed via YOUTUBE and two sets of videos that must be viewed via YOUTUBE.

2. Explanation of the purpose of the class

3. Pretest

4. PowerPoint presentation # 1

5. Video Presentation # 1

6. Posttest

7. PowerPoint presentation # 2

8. Video Presentation # 2

URL and titles of videos should also be viewed via **YouTube.**
There are questions for self-testing and reference materials.
All PowerPoint, videos, and other materials have been chosen to reinforce learning of the signs of ASD and to reinforce effective communication for HCP

PURPOSE

The latest data reported in April 2018 states that the occurrence of Autism Spectrum Disorder (ASD) in the United States is 1:59 children which is an increase from 1:68 reported in the Center for Disease Control (CDC) report of 2010-2012 (Center for Disease Control: Division of Birth Defects, 2018). The CDC has recommended an ideal time of diagnosis for ASD to be between ages of 18 months and 2 years.

Even though research supports a diagnosis of ASD as early as possible, "only 20 percent of U.S. children are diagnosed before the age of 3 yrs." (CDC: Autism and Developmental Disabilities Monitoring Network, 2017a).

A delayed diagnosis of ASD places a child on a trajectory towards responding poorly to intervention services which can interfere with their academic and social success and also places increased stressors on the family. A *high number of low income children* may only be seen in acute situations by an ER physician. In 2005 a study conducted by the Healthcare Cost and Utilization Project in 23 U.S. reported that:

> "One-quarter of all ER visits (55 million) for this data set were children. Children between the ages of 0 and 4 were 2.5 times more likely to make an ER visit than those between ages 5 and 14. The rate of ER visits made by children was 86.1% higher in lower-income communities than the rates in wealthier communities" (Herman & Jackson, 2010, p.896).

There are two *factors, HCP ineffective communication skills and delayed* and/or *obstructed care during ER visits* that support the premise that there is a need for further research and tools aimed at affecting health outcomes of children in the low income communities in positive ways. This is especially important in the health outcomes of low income children who are in the at risk age group for ASD.

In recent years, there have been many scholarly journal articles referring to the imbalance in early diagnosis of ASD between mainstream and low income children, "…there's a big disparity in the degree to which exposure to issues related to autism is 'casually available' in different communities" (Yu, 2010, p.1).

Early diagnosis hinges not only on awareness of signs of ASD by parents and HCP but also on effective communication between parents and HCP. In addressing the contribution of ineffective communication skills of HCP to delayed diagnosis of ASD in low income parents/children scholarly studies support the fact that HCP (specifically physicians) display ineffective communication skills when engaging with those they encounter from low SES groups (Howard, Jacobson and Kripalani, 2013).

Recent studies have revealed that many children of low socio-economic status (SES) are not diagnosed of ASD until school age:

> "…a baseline study conducted by CDC demonstrated that the prevalence of ASD (diagnosis) among low income children aged 3-10 years is highest in children aged 8 yrs" (CDC: Autism and Developmental Disabilities Monitoring Network, 2017b).

Diagnosis of ASD at age of 8yrs. old is far from the recommended age of ASD diagnosis (18-24 months) that the CDC has reported as being ideal. Diagnosis at 8yrs old should be considered an outrage to everyone. It will take a village of HCP to make a positive change in the staggering number of low income children whose diagnosis of ASD are being delayed. *The goal of the training/instruction in this booklet is to present techniques for exchanging and sharing information to promote the internalization of new behaviors by members of a target group, namely Healthcare Providers (HCP) who service low income groups that in time will have a positive affect the health outcomes of low income children at risk for ASD.*

How To Use This Booklet

This is a training program designed to be used a learning tool over and over again.

It is comprised of two sets of PowerPoint slides printed in this book and they may also be

viewed via YouTube and two sets of videos that can only be viewed via YouTube

Explanation of the purpose of the class

Pretest

PowerPoint #1

Video Presentation #1

PowerPoint #2

Video Presentation #2

Posttest

All PowerPoint, videos, and other materials have been chosen to reinforce learning of

the signs of ASD and to reinforce effective communication for HCP

Pretest Questions

1. Which gender is at a high risk for Autism Spectrum Disorder (ASD)?
   a)Boys   b) Girls   c) Both

2. Autistic children like to snuggle with people.
   a)True   b) False

3. Most children on the Autism Spectrum are shy which is why they do not engage in direct eye contact with others but after they get to know someone they will have good eye contact.
   a)True   b) False

4. Many children with ASD display repetitive behavior such as
   a) spinning the wheels of a toy car with their hand over and over
   b) flipping a toy over and over
   c) flapping their hands (shaking)
   d) turning around in circles
   e) all of the above

5. Most children with ASD like to play games with children in their own age group.
   a)True   b) False

PowerPoint slides #1 to #21 are printed in this booklet however you may also use the URL or the title below to locate on **YouTube**

URL:
 https://youtu.be/phcrCXjGzTo

Title:
PowerPoint#1 Recognizing the Signs of Autism Spectrum Disorder Facilitator guide

Introduction PowerPoint #1
The following slides will elaborate on common signs of ASD

- Autism or Autism Spectrum Disorder (ASD) refers to a **broad range of conditions** displayed by challenges.

- It is called a spectrum because each person with autism can have unique strengths and challenges including:

- odd and repetitive behaviors

- impaired speech and nonverbal communication

- lack of social skills

- sensory issues can include aversions to certain, sights, sounds, sensations

Autism Spectrum Disorder
Who is at risk for a delayed diagnosis?
LOW   INCOME   CHILDREN

Why is an early diagnosis important?

Diagnosis after the age of 2yrs (CDC) can have a negative effect on the ability of the child to succeed academically and socially.

**Autism affects an estimated
1 in 59 children in the U.S.**

Some signs of ASD can be detected
in a 4month old baby

- Not cooing
- Not babbling
- Unable to play the peek-a-boo game
- However most signs usually appear by
- age 2 to 3

Classic Sign of ASD # 1
covering ears, usually to loud noise but sounds do not have to be loud...it could be a buzzing or humming sound

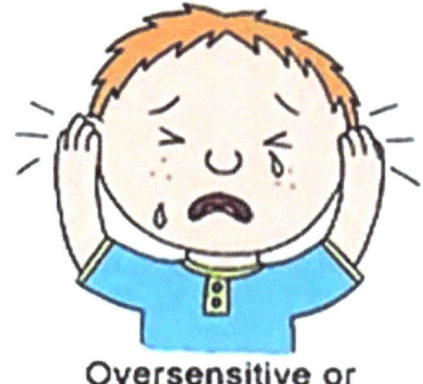

Oversensitive or
undersensitive to sound

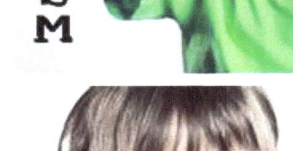

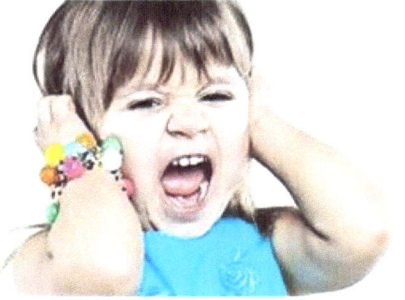

Classic sign of ASD #2
Easily becomes Fixated on Lining up objects or spinning objects

Playing with toys in ways that don't make sense to others

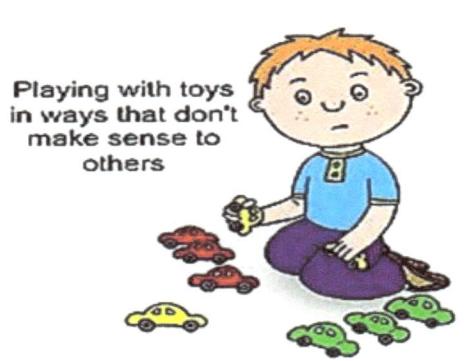
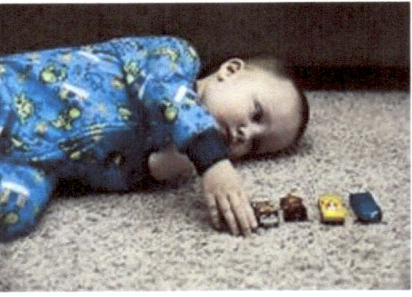
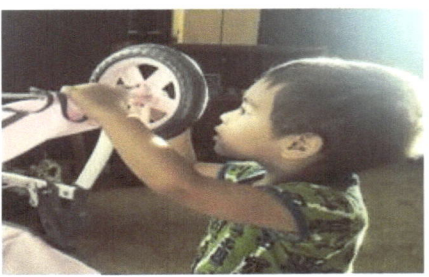

Classic Sign of ASD #3
Inability to interact with socially with others

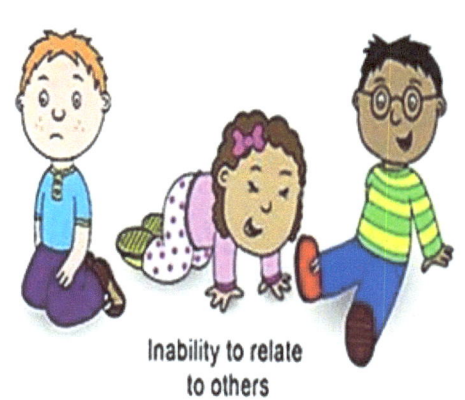

Inability to relate
to others

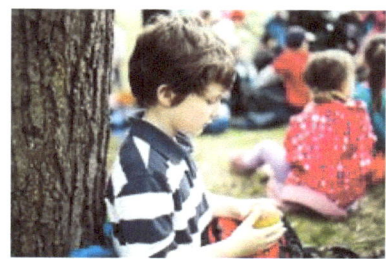

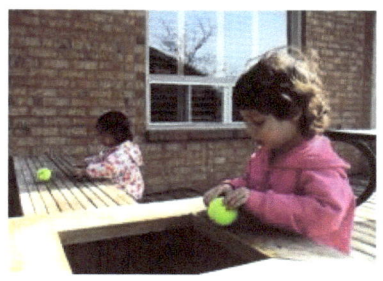

Classic Sign of ASD # 4
Unaware of The Danger of Traffic and Water

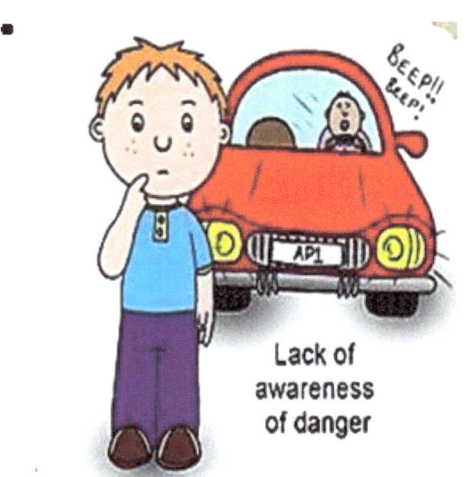

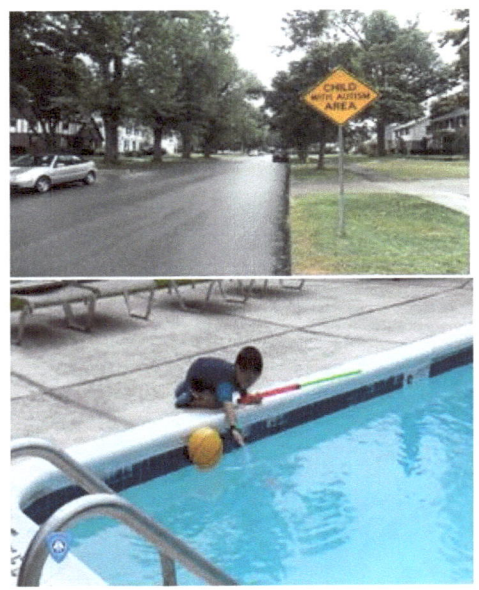

Classic Sign of ASD #5
Wandering

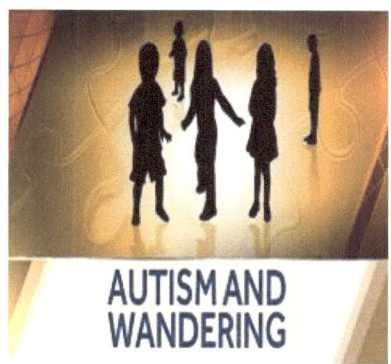

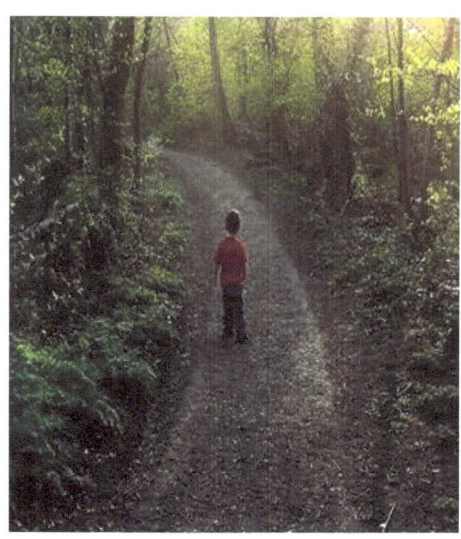

Opportunities for observation of signs of ASD

- "ER visits 86.1% higher in lower-income communities than in wealthier communities" (Herman & Jackson, 2010)

- According to this STUDY the ER is the most likely place to observe LOW INCOME children in the at risk age group for signs of ASD.

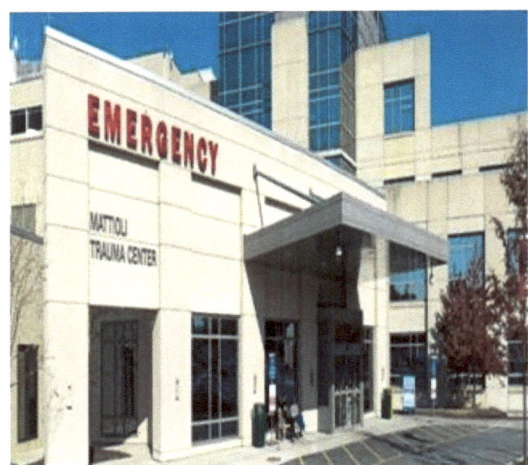

Opportunities for observation of signs of ASD

- **In the ER waiting area children are in a holding pattern**

- **May be EASILY observed as HCP staff are walking in and out of the area.**

- **HCP Knowledge of signs of ASD can help detect abnormal behaviors**

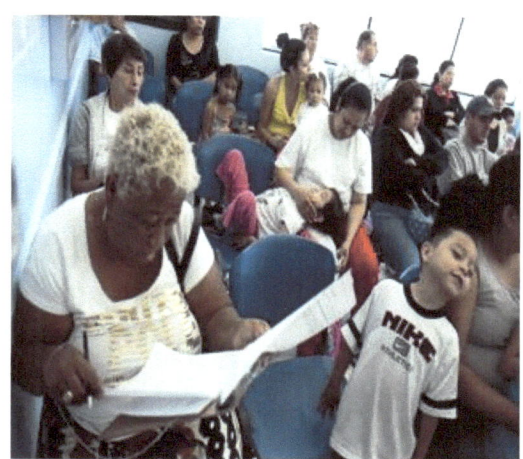

OPPORTUNITIES TO OBSERVE SIGNS OF ASD

- The Certified Nurse Assistant (CNA) in most ER is usually the first to engage with the family

- It is an opportunity to observe any signs of ASD

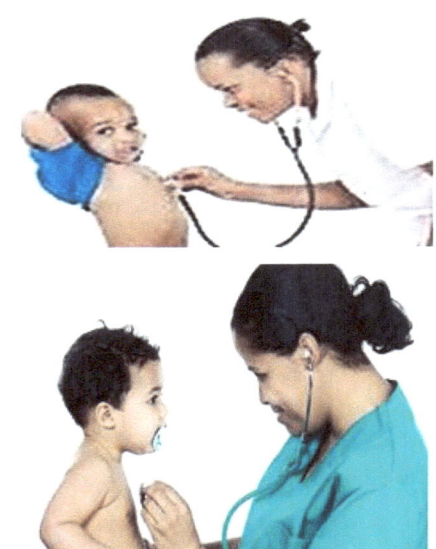

OPPORTUNITIES TO OBSERVE
SIGNS OF ASD

- The Licensed Practical Nurse (LPN) or the Registered Nurse (RN) engages with the family for an assessment

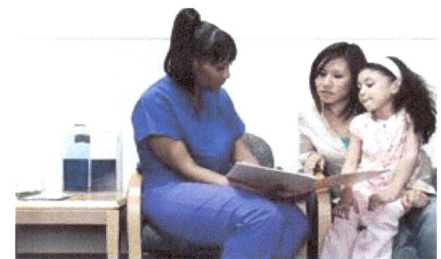

- prime position to ask open ended questions of any signs ASD that can be relayed to the physician

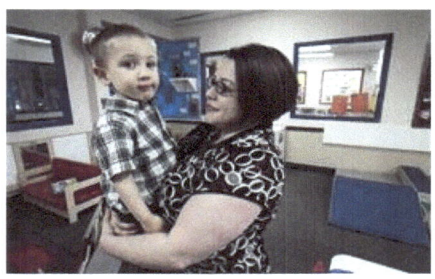

OPPORTUNITIES TO OBSERVE SIGNS OF ASD

- The Emergency room is a very busy place physician have to see patients in a limited amount of time

- The input from the other HCP on any signs or suspicion of ASD helps to guide the ER physician questions and in referring a child for ASD evaluation

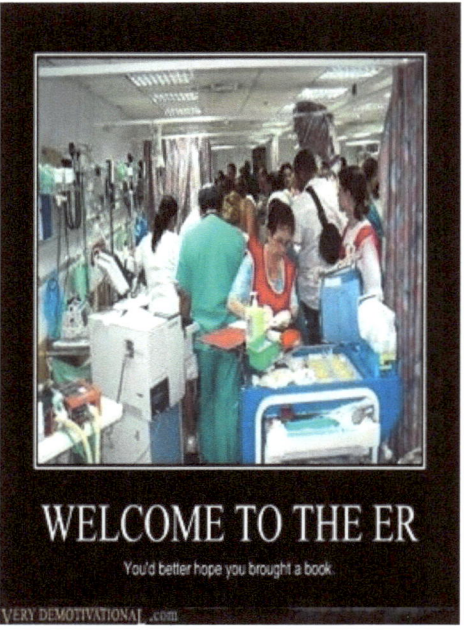

- Relaying observations and suspicions are a key to early diagnosis

  and

- easy to incorporate into a child's visit to the ER…when HCP know the signs

- signs are sparks that call for further observation and for questioning the parent/caregiver about ASD signs even if the child is in the ER for an earache.

OBSERVE AND REPORT

When sitting in the play area, Timmy was **not engaging** with the other children his age

I noticed Timmy **covering his ears** a great deal and the noise in the waiting room was not very loud today

Sarah was **turning around in circles** and staring into space for a long time

HCP can use open ended questions to validate their observations and suspicions

- Ms. Jackson I noticed that Timmy was spinning around in circles in the waiting room, how often have you noticed him doing that?

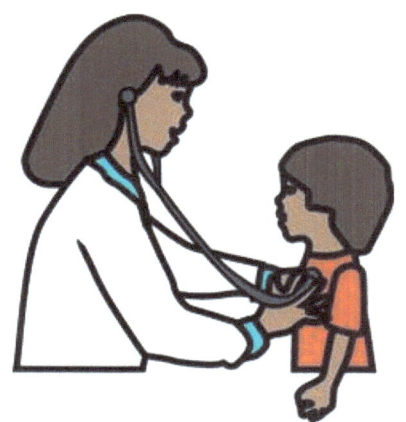

Suspicions Are Enough

- A key to early diagnosis of ASD

- Speak UP !

-

- A diagnosis is a process that <u>starts</u> with a suspicion and a referral.

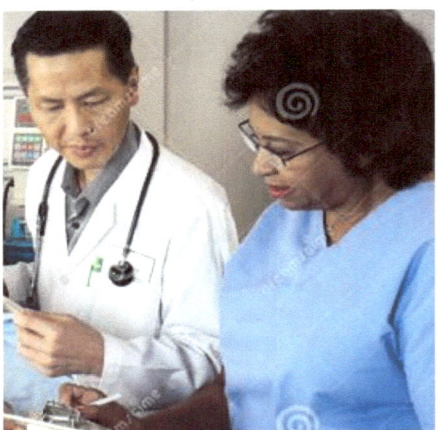

Utilize other family members to aid in getting more information

- Do not hesitate to address a question to a sibling if they are available, they may be more aware of a behavior than the parent.

  Mary when do you see Sarah spin around in circles and how long will she spin?

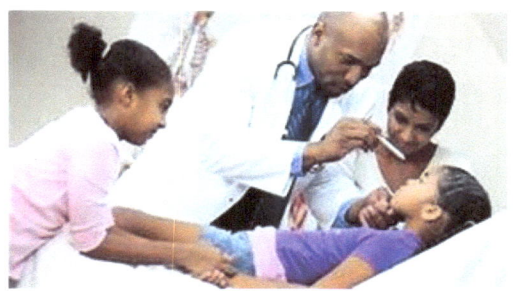

Observations of ASD are easy to pick out from normal behaviors

- Ms. Jones **what kinds of noises have you noticed** cause Timmy to cover his ears ?

- or

- Ms. Jones what has occurred when you notice **Timmy covers his ears.**

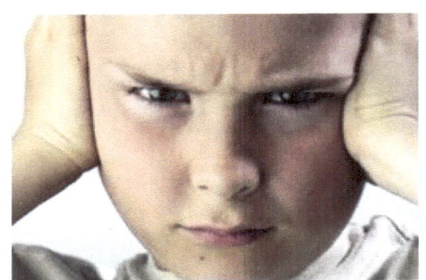

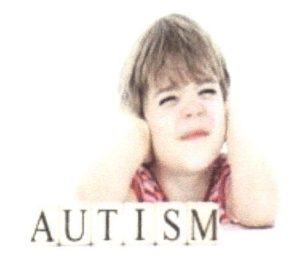

AUTISM

26

Knowledge of signs of ASD may not be as well known in Low income groups for a variety of reasons, language barriers, educational level, culture etc. So HCP should <u>not wait on parents/caregivers</u> to relay information that they may not be aware of…or in denial of…

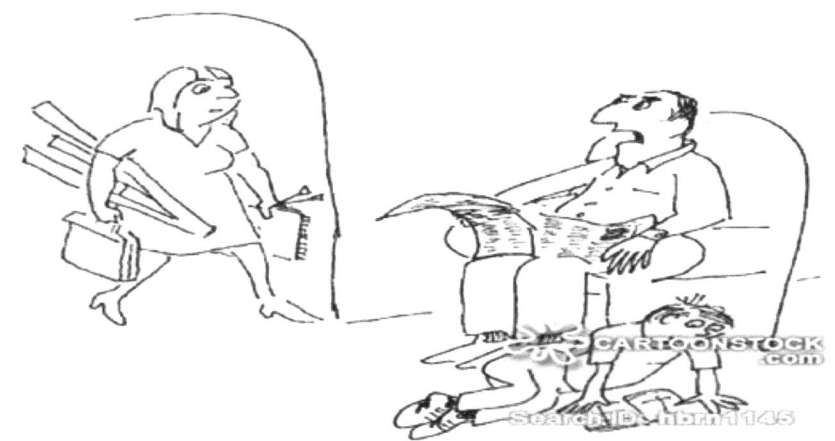

"MABLE, THE DOCTOR SAID THAT TIMMY IS 'AUTISTIC', NOT ARTISTIC."

IT WILL TAKE A MEDICAL VILLAGE TO MAKE A DIFFERENCE

HCP EQUIPPED WITH

1. Effective Communication Skills

2. Knowledge of signs of ASD

3. Use of Open ended Questions

4. Speaking up - Team work
can help reduce the high rate of
delayed diagnosis of ASD in low
income children

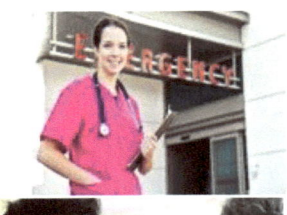

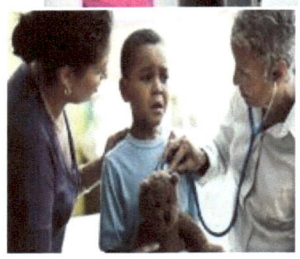

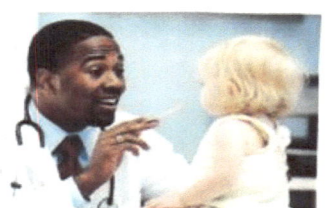

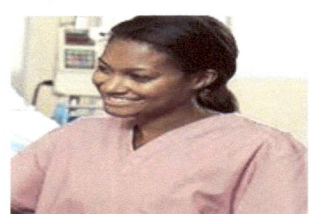

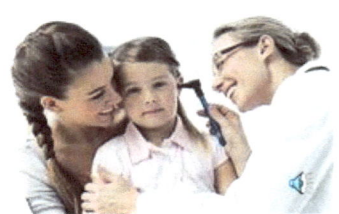

Now that you have read the PowerPoint slides #1 thru #21 the next step is to view the videos 1- 4 via **YOUTUBE** to reinforce the PowerPoint presentation

Video presentation # 1

Video # 1 (2:41)

Why should Healthcare Providers receive training on Autism Spectrum Disorder?

https://youtu.be/h5MpL88fWdo

Video #2 (1:48)

Communicating with Non-verbal Children

https://youtu.be/K5u3phgretk

Video #3 (5:24)

Autism Awareness Video: Diagnostic Criteria for Autism

https://youtu.be/3w1c4sF4ZTg

Video # 4 (1:51)

Early signs of Autism: Stimming (play in mute mode)

https://youtu.be/IdDulavkBOo

PowerPoint presentation #2
Effective Communication Techniques

Remember you may also use YouTube to view these slides

URL
https://youtu.be/i8G4-EhpMkg

Or

Title:

PowerPoint #2 Recognizing the signs of Autism Spectrum Disorder Effective Communication Techniques

Introduction
HCP must be aware of barriers
Early diagnosis of ASD in Marginalized children hinges on awareness of signs and on effective communication between parents and HCP

Many journal articles refer to the imbalance in early diagnosis of ASD between mainstream and marginalized children

"There's a big disparity in the degree to which exposure to issues related to autism is casually available in different communities..." (Yu, 2017).

Do Most HCP Recognize the negative Impact of ineffective communication skills on marginalized groups?

- One well known study concluded in that participating residents "did not use positive communication skills with any consistency and overestimated their ability to communicate clearly to those with low health literacy." (Howard, et.al, 2013)

32

Why is it important for HCP to utilize effective communication with marginalized groups?

- ***Ineffective*** *communication skills* used by HCP is a known factor in negative health outcomes (Jördis, et al., 2014)

- Delayed diagnosis of ASD is a negative health outcome in marginalized children

◁

Nonverbal clues   1

When a patient/parent is nodding and giving a blank look this may be the first indication that they do Not understand what is being relayed to them.
(Knapp & Hall, 2008)

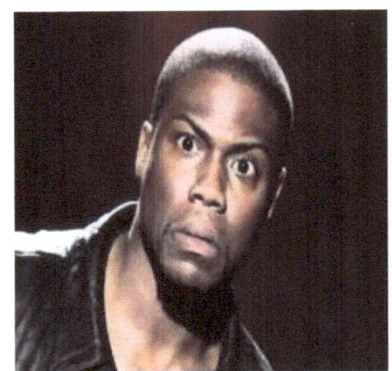

Nonverbal Clues   2
a confused facial look

- Some Physicians with an accent may be difficult to understand by low income patients/parents who are not accustom to hearing languages other than their own.

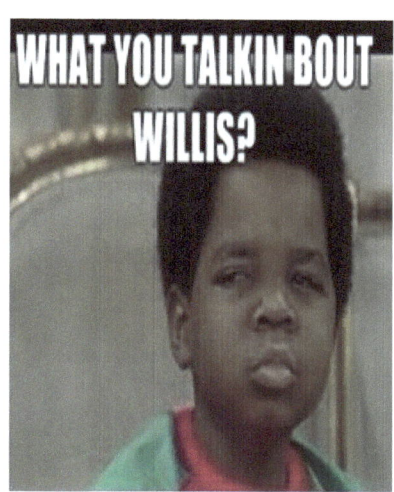

- Physicians must become more aware that their accent and/or use of medical terminology can short circuit the flow of information to a patient.

Nonverbal Clues   3
Medical Jargon

- Some patients/parents may have trouble understanding the health information and medical terminology HCP regularly use

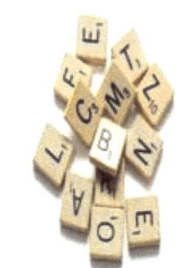

- Medical jargon has been described as "a second language used by HCP to shorten and ease communication

  … medical shorthand can cause confusion and diminish understanding between HCP and patient." (Graham & Brookey, 2008)

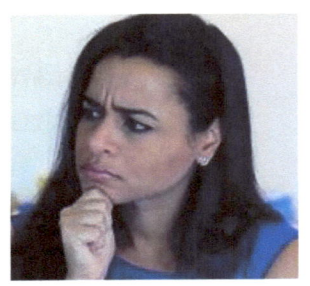

Medical jargon can be a communication barrier between HCP and Patients

- **"Overuse of medical terminology can inhibit patients' ability to filter out facts critical to their decision-making process. To promote health literacy, the use of medical terminology and acronyms in patient/parent encounters is discouraged."** (Killian & Coletti,2017)

- **In the study mentioned earlier the participating residents used an average of 2 medical terms (jargon) per minute**

  and

- **less than a 1/4 of them used the teach-back method when communicating with marginalized groups** (Howard et.al, 2013)

THE TEACH-BACK METHOD

- The teach-back method is a way for HCP to explain information clearly by asking the patient to explain in their own words what was relayed to them.

  This demonstrates their understanding.

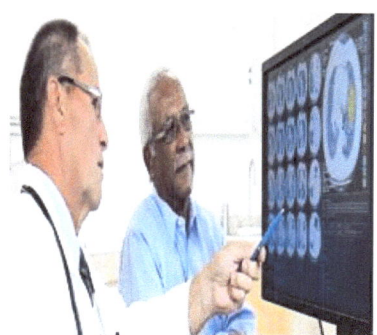

- "The teach-back method helps to educate patients/parents with low health literacy and improve their comprehension of health information" (Porter,et.al 2015)

WHY USE OPEN-ENDED QUESTIONS ?

Open-ended questions can not be answered with

a yes or a no

"They encourage the patient/parent to reflect on their problem, their pain, their symptoms." (Maynard & Heritage, 2005)

Effective Communication Weapon 1
Ask Open ended questions

- **Can I help you?**

  Is a closed ended question because it can be answered with a yes or no

- **What brings you to the hospital today?**

  Requires elaboration and specifics

Effective Communication Weapon 2
GOOD EYE CONTACT

- Being a more effective communicator

  can actually be as simple as maintaining

  eye contact

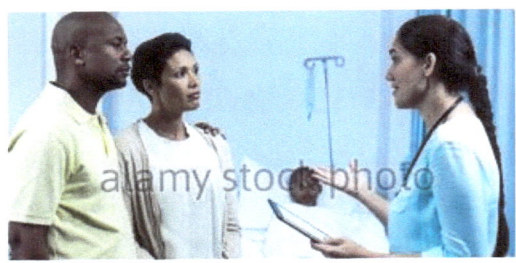

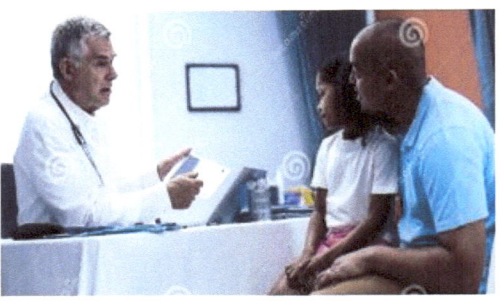

Effective Communication Weapon 3
Empathy

Empathy is one part
Emotional awareness
and
at least two parts
body language

**HCP should position
their body to appear
attentive and interested**.

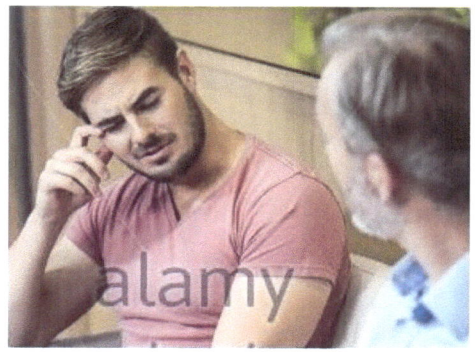

Effective Communication Weapon 4
Smile

- A **genuine smile** can encourage feelings of warmth and safety.

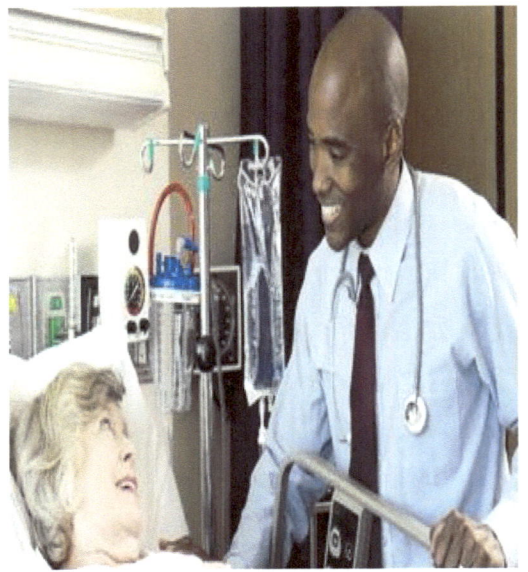

Effective communication Weapon 5
Avoidance of Bias

- HCP should **be aware** of any bias that may have.

- **Unrecognized bias may affect communication and the care of patients.**

- Dislikes or stereotypes should **not be a factor** in care of individuals.

- **Respect, courtesy** and **tone** can help eliminate biased communication.

Effective communication and knowledge of signs of ASD may positively impact the high rate of delayed diagnosis of ASD in marginalized children

HCP acting as a team observing and reporting signs of ASD
HCP Utilizing open-ended questions, good eye contact and a genuine smile may help parents to divulge more information about their child's abnormal behaviors.
HCP's empathy and understanding of the unique health concerns and disparities common to marginalized groups may motivate the HCP to become more proactive in looking for signs of ASD and in asking more questions of the parents of at risk children.

Video Presentation #2

(The following videos reinforce the importance of effective communication between HCP and parents of low income children and the importance of communication between HCP staff with each other)

Video # 5 (3:16)

An inside look at one of Chicago area's busy trauma centers

https://youtu.be/IdDulavkBOo

Most emergency rooms in low income communities are very busy.   Doctors and nurses have to switch gears from patient to patient and have little time to focus on any symptoms other the acute problem the patient may be having at the time seen.
This is one of the main reasons that when it comes to ASD
all eyes need to be on deck for signs and be proactive in reporting any suspicions.

Video #6 (4:57)

The importance of communication in healthcare: The time is now!

https://youtu.be/b7YwrHNylTg

This video by the American Academy on communication in healthcare explains the need to improve communication and the importance of team work among HCP.

Video #7(2:52)

Poor Nurse Communication

https://youtu.be/bwqwFCxVhEY

This is an exaggeration of poor communication skills

Video #8 (3:01)

Good Nurse Communication

https://youtu.be/Wu9LxyVDFYE

This is an example of an encounter that is a positive display of good communication. The nurse was non-judgmental, forth coming with vitally helpful information and seemed knowledgeable and genuinely caring.

Video #9 (1:40)

Recognizing and challenging unconscious bias: Everyone matters

https://youtu.be/F8JKUCvGJ7I

We need to be more aware of our thoughts and the bias we project onto others

Video #10 (1:05)

Bad patient and Doctor interaction

https://youtu.be/2kLDm0rAAZ8

The patient is not an object that one can talk over and negatively about.
This manner of interaction lacks empathy and is very disrespectful.

Video #11 (2:50)

Good patient interaction

https://youtu.be/laZ7sP8QnDw

Key words: Respectful
            Non-judgmental
            Informative

Video # 12   (2:58)

Physician Communication: Model of Communication in Healthcare

https://youtu.be/phkuG_FqPF4

Perspectives by some physicians in a communication class at the Cleveland Clinic on the benefits of post medical school training on effective communication skills.

Post test

1. Autism happens in all socio economic, ethnic and racial groups but girls are most likely to suffer.
    a) True   b) False

2. Autism is called Autism Spectrum Disorder (ASD) because the symptoms vary from person to person.
    a) True   b) False

3. All children on the Autism Spectrum whether mild or severe are challenged in areas of communication and social skills.
    a)   True   b) False

4. The CDC recommended age for diagnosis of ASD is during the first year of school around age 5-6.
    a)   True   b) False

5. Red flags that an infant could have Autism may be detected
    as early as 4 months old if the baby does not

    a) Maintain eye contact
    b) Respond to games of peek a boo
    c) Coo and babble
    d) All of the above

ANSWER KEY

PRE TEST
1.   A
2.   B
3.   B
4.   E
5.   B

POST TEST

1.   False
2.   True
3.   True
4.   False
5.   D (all of the above)

References

Autism Spectrum Disorder Fact Sheet (2015). Patient-Caregiver Education

Retrieved from

https://www.ninds.nih.gov/Disorders/Patient-Caregiver-Education/Fact-

Sheets/Autism-Spectrum-Disorder-Fact-Sheet

Bombeke, K., Van Roosbroeck, S., De Winter, B., Debaene, L., Schol, S., Van Hal, G.,

et al. (2011). Medical students trained in communication skills show a decline in

patient-centered attitudes: An observational study comparing two cohorts during

clinical clerkships. Patient Education and Counseling, 84.

https://doi.org/10.3109/0142159X.2012.670320

Center for Disease Control, (2018). Autism data and Statistics/birth defects.

Retrieved from

https://www.cdc.gov/ncbddd/autism/data.html

Center for Disease Control, (2017). Autism Spectrum Disorder: Monitoring Network.

Retrieved from

https://www.cdc.gov/ncbddd/autism/monitoring network.html

Center for Disease Control, (2018). Screening and Diagnosis for Healthcare Providers.

Retrieved from

https://www.cdc.gov/ncbddd/autism/hcp-screening.html

Diagnostic and Statistical Manual of Mental Disorders, 5th, Edition. (2013). DSM-5.

American Psychiatric Association Publishing, Arlington County, VA

doi/book/10.1176/appi.books.9780890425596

Drotar, D. (2009). Physician behavior in the care of pediatric chronic

   illness: Association with health outcomes and treatment adherence.

   Journal of Developmental & Behavioral Pediatrics, 30.

   doi: 10.1080/10410236.2011.616632

   https://www.ncbi.nlm.nih.gov/pmc/articles/PMC3413374/

Freed G., Dunham K., Switalski K., Jones M., & McGuinness, G. (2009). Research

   Advisory Committee of the American Board of Pediatrics, Pediatric fellows:

   perspectives on training and future scope of practice. Pediatrics, 123.

    https://www.ncbi.nlm.nih.gov/pubmed/19088243

Graham, S., Brookey, J., 2008. Do Patients Understand?

   Permanente Journal. 12

   https://www.ncbi.nlm.nih.gov/pmc/articles/PMC3037129/#i1552-5775-12-3-67-

Herman, A. & Jackson, P. (2010). Empowering Low-Income Parents with Skills

   to Reduce Excess Pediatric Emergency Room and Clinic Visits through a

   Tailored Low Literacy Training Intervention.

   Journal of Health Communication, 15.

   doi: 10.1080/10810730.2010.522228

Howard, T., Jacobson, K. & Kripalani, S. (2013). Doctor Talk: Physicians' Use of Clear

   Verbal Communication. Journal of Health Communication. 18.

   doi: 10.1080/10810730.2012.757398

Jordis, M.,Christalle,E., Muller, E.,Harter,M., Dirmaier, J.,Scholl, I. (2014).

Measurement of Physician-Patient Communication-A Systematic Review.

doi: 10.1371/journal.pone.0112637

Retrieved from

https://www.ncbi.nlm.nih.gov/pmc/articles/PMC4273948/#pone.

Killian, L. & Coletti, 2017. The Role of Universal Health Literacy Precautions in

Minimizing "Medspeak" and Promoting Shared Decision Making.

Journal of Ethics.

https://journalofethics.ama-assn.org/article/role-universal-health-literacy-

Knapp, M. & Hall, J. (2008). Nonverbal communication in human communication

(6th ed.). Thomson Wadsworth. Belmont, CA

Levinson, W., Lesser, C., & Epstein, R. (2010). Developing physician communication

skills for patient-centered care. Health Affairs, 29.

doi: 10.1377/hlthaff.2009.0450.

Retrieved from

https://www.ncbi.nlm.nih.gov/pubmed/20606179

Maynard, D. & Heritage, J. (2005). Conversation analysis, doctor-patient interaction

and medical communication. Medical Education, 39

Porter, K., Chen, Y., Estabrooks, P., Noel, L., Bailey,A., Zoellner, J., (2015).

Using Teach-Back to Understand Participant Behavioral Self-Monitoring Skills

across Health Literacy Level and Behavioral Condition.

doi: [10.1016/j.jneb.2015.08.012]

https://www.ncbi.nlm.nih.gov/pmc/articles/PMC4715922/

Swedlund,M., Schumacher,J., Young,H., & Cox, E. (2012). Effect of

Communication Style and Physician–Family Relationships on Satisfaction with

Pediatric Chronic Disease Care. Health Communication, 27.

doi: 10.1080/10410236.2011.616632

https://www.ncbi.nlm.nih.gov/pmc/articles/PMC

U.S. Preventive Service Task Force (2016).

Retrieved from

www.uspreventiveservicestaskforce.org/Page/Document/UpdateSummaryFinal/au

tism-spectrum-disorder-in-young-children-screening

Wilkin, H., Cohen, E., &Tannebaum, M. (2012). How Low-Income Residents

Decide Between Emergency and Primary Health Care for Non-Urgent Treatment,

The Howard Journal of Communications, 23.

doi:10.1080/10646175.2012.66772

Yu, B. (2017). How Do We Better Identify and Support Minorities with Autism?

ASHA Leader. 22

Retrieved from

http://leader.pubs.asha.org/article.aspx?articleid=2615522

Zandbelt, L., Smets, E., Oort, F., Godfried, M., de Haes, H. (2007). Medical

specialists'patient-centered communication and patient-reported outcomes.

Retrieved from

https://www.ncbi.nlm.nih.gov/pubmed/1749

What are early signs of autism?

The timing and severity of autism's early signs vary widely. Some infants show hints BY 4 MONTHS OLD…

In others, symptoms become obvious as late as age 2 or 3.

The following "red flags" may indicate a child is at risk for an autism spectrum disorder.

6 months

•Few or no big smiles or other warm, joyful and engaging expressions.

•Limited or no eye contact.

9 months

•Little or no back-and-forth sharing of sounds, smiles or other facial expressions

12 months

•Little or no babbling

•Little or no back-and-forth gestures such as pointing, showing, reaching or waving

•Little or no response to name.

16 months

•Very few or no words.

24 months

•Very few or no meaningful, two-word phrases (not including imitating or repeating)

Signs At any age

• Loss of previously acquired speech, babbling or social skills

• Avoidance of eye contact

• Persistent preference for solitude

• Difficulty understanding other people's feelings

• Delayed language development

• Persistent repetition of words or phrases (echolalia)

• Resistance to minor changes in routine or surroundings

• Restricted interests

• Repetitive behaviors (flapping, rocking, spinning, etc.)

• Unusual and intense reactions to sounds, smells, tastes, textures, lights and/or color

Stimming is a hallmark sign of ASD.

Actions such as head banging, sitting on the ground and twirling over and over or hand-flapping are classic forms of stimming, but there are many expressions of stimming

They include

•Staring at objects — especially anything with lights or movement

•Gazing off into space

•Blinking repeatedly

•Looking out of the corner of your eyes

•Flipping lights on and off repeatedly

•Random humming, shrieking, or making other noises

•Finger snapping, tapping or putting your hands over your ears.

•Tapping on ears or objects

•Covering and uncovering ears

•Repeating words or phrases including lines from a TV show, songs, or any other kind of repetitive verbalization

•Scratching or rubbing your skin in a repetitive manner.

•Any kind repetitive movement: spinning, pacing, twirling

•Tasting or licking — including thumb sucking, finger sucking, or tasting something one wouldn't normally taste

•Unusual or inappropriate smelling or sniffing

When a person with ASD feels anxious or overwhelmed or uncomfortable in a social situation, STIMMING can be their way of calming their mind.

While stress can bring on stimming as a response, ironically the opposite is true as well. For instance, when a person is bored it becomes a way to deal with thoughts and feelings that have no place to go. An unoccupied mind and idle body isn't necessarily in a state of calm; in ASD it can create a sense of tension or panic.

The information in this booklet may also be found on Kindle ebook.

This information may be copied and disseminated anyone even if they are not a HCP.

The information is for learning purposes; the more people view it and become equipped with the knowledge of signs of ASD the better off we as a society will be.

Commercials have been aired over the years regarding the signs of a heart attack and stroke which has been a benefit to many lay people.

My prayer is for the signs of ASD to become automatic for a far greater number of people so that the prevalence of delayed diagnosis in all children becomes rare.

www.ingramcontent.com/pod-product-compliance
Lightning Source LLC
Chambersburg PA
CBHW050800180526
45159CB00004B/1502